Safe and Effective?
Why Medical Freedom is Worth Fighting For

Katelyn McCormack, RN, BSN, PHN

Contents

Preface

I have watched people's perception of me change in an instant. Immediately, I was no longer intelligent. Immediately, my parenting skills were questioned. Immediately, I was crazy. These were friends and family who already knew me and understood that I love my children more than anyone in the world. But in an instant, because of one thing I said, their respect for me vanished.

I have lost friends, and at times I have lost faith. Never in my decision, but in humanity itself. I have listened to a family member belittle my intelligence, I have listened to a relative berate my family values, and I have watched my friend turn her back on me. The reason I lost faith was that no one was willing to listen. No one wanted an explanation, no one wanted to take the time to hear why, or to read the books or research papers I offered. With extreme arrogance, they just assumed that they knew more and never considered the possibility that I had read more studies, had stayed up more nights reading, talking, dissecting, and processing the information from both sides.

The hardest part of all, they assumed they knew what was best for my kids. Whether they intended to or not, they questioned my ability to parent and protect my children. They

1

assumed a role they never earned. It is with this broken heart, I share my challenges and findings in the hope that I am able to help others avoid the anguish of someone else's ignorance.

The conversation on vaccinating versus not vaccinating has become so volatile that it is no longer a conversation at all. As a Registered Nurse, licensed Public Health Nurse, and someone who has worked in healthcare for over a decade, I have seen and heard how these "conversations" go. Either you accept the pre-scripted narrative, or you say nothing at all. PubMed is not referenced and studies are not quoted. I have spent 5 years becoming an expert, reviewing the literature, starting the dialogue, and questioning everything. I have spoken at conferences, universities, and attended meetings with elected officials. With every conversation comes a chance to promote acceptance, a chance to open a dialogue that may never have occurred, and the chance to open someone's mind to an idea they never considered.

Through my personal struggles as a mother, sister, daughter, nurse, and friend to discuss vaccines, I saw a common thread: we all want our children to be healthy. In this book I will share with you the reader, especially those of you that are considering utilizing vaccines, the new reality that vaccines might not be as safe or effective as we were led to believe. This is not what you will read in pamphlets at your doctor's office. This information is not shared on television, and most distressingly, you may not even hear this from your own sister. She may be hiding what she knows because she, like many others, does not want to rock the boat. We all want to get along, to be healthy, and to feel connected with our community. I ask you to consider that by finding out the truth and supporting each other, we can possibly be more connected and healthier than ever.

I write to the parents making the tough decisions, and I write to the friends and family of those individuals. Hear me well. We have not become less intelligent, our love for our children has not waned, and our instincts have not broken. We are still the loving, caring parents we have always been. Remember this as you read.

Introduction

This book was written to help shed light on some of the most challenging aspects of sharing a personal decision. It is often easy to get tongue-tied when having a discussion about vaccinations. The conversation often gets heated very quickly, rash judgments get made, emotions take over, and listening and respect go out the window. The purpose of this text is to empower individuals to navigate these difficult conversations by having a tool that can ease the burden of a challenging discussion. It is a resource meant to deliver the shorthand version of the many thoughts and talking points one has heard and processed, leading to the decision one ultimately makes for a child and family.

As with any discussion, there is more than one side and more than one perspective. Simply put, there are two main camps to this discussion: pro medical freedom and pro vaccine compliance. Societal slang refers to these groups as anti or pro-vax, respectively. It is important to understand the mission of individuals unfairly labeled anti-vax and why using this terminology is not appropriate.

Advocates for medical freedom stand on the principle that you are the only one who should have control over your body. No one, including government officials, should have the right or power to control what happens to your body. Bodily autonomy is of the utmost importance.

The term "anti-vax" is inappropriate for this discussion in that it assumes medical freedom advocates believe a child should never be vaccinated. This is simply not true. Advocates fundamentally believe no one, other than oneself, has control over another's body. This belief extends to not denying others access to an intervention they feel is right for their family.

Individuals who are pro vaccine compliance typically believe that everyone should be required to receive all vaccinations for the benefit of the greater good. This idea does not consider an individual's rights or health history. It places the perceived benefit of society over the wellness of the individual.

Lastly, it is important to take into account that the majority of individuals who are pro medical freedom are individuals who initially complied with the vaccination schedule. They are not anti-vax, they are ex-vax. All vaccine adverse reactions are due to vaccine compliant parents. People typically don't choose this path, it is one that unfortunately finds them.

Chapter 1
Foundational Knowledge For A Vaccination Discussion

This topic is very complex. This book will do its best to simplify the moving parts, key points, and major players so we can be on the same page during our discussion. This approach is to show you that decisions are not made off one idea or dispute. Decisions are the result of synthesizing many different ideas, rationales, as well as moral, ethical, and scientific research studies. Knowing all of the players helps to demonstrate why there is a foundation for reasonable doubt and to let you see the breadth of information behind a topic that most do not yet fully understand.

As with all medical interventions, vaccination being just one of them, individuals have the right to be fully informed regarding the risks, benefits, and alternative options to the intervention. Having all of this information prior to the intervention is what is referred to as informed consent. Up until recently, it has been commonly understood by the medical community, and beyond, that we all have the right to be informed and then have the ability to give consent.

In order to give consent, one must fully understand the context of what they are considering. The current vaccine schedule is drastically different now than in previous generations. In the late 1950's, 3 vaccines, covering 5 diseases were recommended (Offit, 2019). In 1986, a typical child received vaccines for 8 diseases totaling 12 shots by the age of 18. Currently, most children receive at least 54 doses covering 16 diseases (CDC, 2019)!

The vaccine schedule is changing swiftly with more vaccines being studied every year. The vaccine industry has had tremendous growth over the last couple decades creating a dense schedule. Knowing how the industry operates will help shine light on the current schedule and how its rapid expansion came to be.

Chapter 2
Vaccine Industry

The vaccine industry is obviously a major player in this discussion. Vaccines are manufactured by pharmaceutical companies like Merck, Pfizer, Sanofi, GlaxoSmithKline, or Novartis and currently make up an almost 60 BILLION dollar industry (Mikulic, 2019). This figure has almost doubled since 2014. Once a vaccine has been brought to the market, The Centers for Disease Control and Prevention (CDC) use the guidelines from the Advisory Committee on Immunization Practices (ACIP) to add the new vaccine to the schedule.

According to the *New York Times*, there is a tremendous amount of conflict of interest between these manufacturers and the organizations promoting the use of such products (Harris, 2009). A report showed that "64 percent of the advisers had potential conflicts of interest that were never identified or were left unresolved by the centers" and "Most of the experts who served on advisory panels in 2007 to evaluate vaccines for flu and cervical cancer had potential conflicts that were never resolved, the report said. Some were legally barred from considering the issues but did so anyway" (Harris, 2009). Notably, 2007 was a very important year for experts to weigh in on the HPV vaccine, as it was FDA approved only the year before.

An interesting point about the vaccine industry is that there is no liability. Liability for vaccine manufacturers was suspended by the government in 1986 due to the high cost of defending vaccines in court (Congress, 1986). If there is a vaccine reaction, injury, or death, one cannot sue the vaccine manufacturer. Individuals must go to the United States Court of Federal Claims and submit a claim to The National Vaccine Injury Compensation Program.

Additionally, proceedings do not contain discovery, making this very different from a traditional court. There is no sharing of information between parties before the "trial," so previously known information does not have to be shared. Previous trial information is thus not used in subsequent trials, meaning everyone starts at square one. After the trial is done and if the individual is awarded restitution, neither the vaccine manufacturer nor the administering physician pay, but rather the money comes from the tax-funded Vaccine Injury Compensation Trust Fund (Health Resources & Services Administration, 2019). Seventy-five cents is collected from every vaccine to fund this program. Yes, vaccinations have *known* risks, and the cost of these risks is built into the purchasing price.

Chapter 3
National Vaccine Injury Compensation Program (VICP)

As just mentioned, the VICP is what is commonly referred to as "vaccine court." According to the CDC, the VICP was created in 1986, after the cost of lawsuits against vaccine manufacturers and health care providers threatened to cause vaccine shortages. So much time and money were being spent trying to defend their products in court that manufacturers were going to have to slow production, which would possibly reduce U.S. vaccination rates. This was thought to be a public health threat, prompting the U.S. government to take on all liability relating to vaccines.

For some, this sounds like a great solution. However, it means there are no checks and balances to the quality of the product being brought to market. If there is a "bad" batch, no one is at fault for that. If a doctor accidentally gives a live virus vaccine to an immunocompromised child, which is a known contraindication, the doctor is not responsible. However, if an anesthesiologist accidentally gives that same child the wrong drug during surgery, he is responsible for that action. Removing the liability and responsibility to practice safe medicine and manufacturing practices can have huge impacts on the quality of the products and care being delivered.

As of February 1, 2018, VICP has paid 3.8 BILLION in claims, even though it is estimated by the U.S. Department of Health and Human Services (Ross & Klompas, 2011) that fewer than 1% of injuries ever get reported. Do the math and think about how much money would need to be paid if 100% of injuries were reported. Why are they not reported? Let's look now at how vaccine injuries get reported through a separate program called the Vaccine Adverse Event Reporting System (VAERS).

Chapter 4
VAERS Information

VAERS stands for the Vaccine Adverse Event Reporting System and is a program co-managed by both the CDC and the FDA, which are agencies of the U.S. Department of Health and Human Services. According to their website, it is a passive reporting system that is useful for detecting unusual or unexpected patterns of adverse event reporting that might indicate a possible safety problem with a vaccine.

On the surface, this program sounds great. However, in actuality, it is not as impressive as one would like to believe. The CDC composed a document called "VAERS Table of Reportable Events Following Vaccination," which details the reactions providers are mandated to report. In addition to these complications, providers are mandated to report any adverse reaction that is listed on the vaccine package insert as a contraindication to an additional dose of the vaccine. This document is important because it dictates that only a few (already documented) conditions are to be reported. This is a significant limiting factor in finding additional complications associated with new vaccinations because they are not to be reported.

This is not to say that parents cannot report new complications, but if people responsible for our safety are not required to report all adverse reactions, then they are not looking out for the greater good. The CDC simply encourages reporting of additional adverse events and also only encourages reporting administration errors. This means if a provider accidentally administers the wrong vaccine, too many vaccines or expired vaccines, they are only "encouraged" to report!

Which brings us back to the point, neither physicians nor vaccine manufacturers are responsible for their actions or products. The liability is absorbed by the U.S. government and paid for by the previously mentioned taxes added on to all vaccines.

When the CDC leans on VAERS as an additional safety measure, yet injury reporting, known as post-market surveillance, is not a requirement, it makes for a very broken system. To provide greater insight on how limited these reporting requirements are, let's look at the actual "Table of Injuries." This will unveil two things: first, vaccines DO have known adverse reactions, and second, the required reporting system is VERY limited.

Chapter 5
Table Of Injuries

The Table of Injuries is a chart that lists all vaccines and known adverse reactions associated with that specific vaccine. There is also a column that notates the time period in which the adverse reaction may have occurred. The table was created solely for the purposes of receiving compensation under the Vaccine Injury Compensation Program (VICP) discussed above.

In order to be eligible to take your claim to the VICP, it must first be already documented on the Table of Injuries and fall within all parameters listed. The document has very specific guidelines and is very limited on what it will acknowledge.

For example, for the Polio vaccine, the Table of Injuries only lists paralytic polio, vaccine-strain polio viral infection, anaphylaxis, shoulder injury related to vaccine administration, and vasovagal syncope. Obviously, these are awful complications and reporting should be required. However, if you have a reaction not listed in the Table of Injuries, then it doesn't need to be reported. Let's say you have multiple seizures immediately post-vaccination, which is listed for other vaccines, it does not need to be reported. Maybe hundreds of people are having seizures but because they don't need to be reported, the Table will never be expanded.

Here is the process if you are "lucky" enough to fit the mold already created. Your child receives the MMR vaccine and has a reaction where he is screaming uncontrollably for hours. You take him to the hospital to learn the reaction is encephalitis, which is a swelling of the brain that can lead to temporary or permanent brain damage. The family spends days in the hospital during which they do some research and find out about VAERS, the adverse event reporting system. The mom then reports the reaction to VAERS.

After this, she goes on to learn about the Table of Injuries and discovers her son's reaction is listed for the appropriate vaccine within the predetermined timeline. Now she is eligible to pursue the VICP for compensation relating to her son's reaction and lifelong injury costs. It takes months to years, attorney fees, and countless hours, all of which she needs to work on and pay for while coping with the new reality of caring for a brain-injured child. Not only is it physically and mentally challenging, but she carries the guilt of knowing that this situation could have been prevented. Why didn't she know about this reaction beforehand? Would she still have done it if she knew? She will never have answers to these questions because just like millions of other parents, she never thought she needed to question the system. She didn't know there were risks, a Table of Injuries, a payout system or countless other parents who can't share their stories because of the guilt or social ridicule of speaking up about vaccine damage.

Instead of having the option to fully give consent, she was awarded what the government thought was the cost of the burden. A dollar amount was put on the life of her child and the lifelong hardship associated with his trauma. This woman's son was unfortunately sacrificed for the government's goal of the greater good. His brain injury was excusable in their minds because the rest of the kids around him were not exposed to the measles virus that he never even carried in the first place.

Chapter 6
Herd Immunity

The story above transitions us to the topic of herd immunity. This is one of the most common arguments for vaccination. Many people support mandated vaccination because they feel it keeps the community healthier as a whole. This opinion is based on something called herd immunity. It is the idea that diseases will not spread through a population if a certain percentage of the population is immune to the disease (typically believed to be 95%). While this would be good in theory, the idea of herd immunity has a few crucial flaws.

First, certain pathogens are always evolving and changing, often known as strain migration. This is when the virus changes or mutates in order to survive the current environment. It can be seen in the need for an annual flu vaccine. Every year a new flu vaccine is developed. We use expert scientists to take an educated guess as to which strains are going to cause the highest amount of disease that year and make the vaccine accordingly. The efficacy is not known until after we administer it to the population and see how well it does.

Also, the strains are known to mutate (antigenic drift) during the season, making the vaccine less effective over time as the mutations occur (CDC, 2019). Bacteria and viruses want to survive, just as people do, so they adapt and change in order to do so. We have also seen this phenomenon with other vaccines such as HPV and Pneumococcal disease.

The first HPV vaccine protected against the 4 most common strains of HPV responsible for cervical cancer. After the vaccine had been implemented, additional strains started to become problematic so a new vaccine was released. Additional strains had to be added that were not originally problematic, but due to the new environment, they became more dangerous.

The same phenomenon occurred with the Pneumococcal vaccine, which started protecting against 7 strains, then was upped to 13 strains and now even has a 23 serotype option for high-risk individuals. The most prevalent strains change, making it necessary to update the vaccine to encompass more strains that are becoming more prevalent over time. However, there is also a lag time between identifying strain migration and updated vaccine manufacturing so we will always be somewhat behind the curve. Even if every individual is getting vaccinated, there is still disease risk from the strains not in the vaccine.

Second, it assumes that the efficacy of a vaccination is very high. This may be true, but for a very short time. Let's consider Pertussis as this is a very feared disease among babies and has a large vaccination campaign. The CDC recommends a pertussis vaccine that is a combination vaccine for diphtheria (D), tetanus

(T) and acellular pertussis (aP). It is recommended for babies as young as 2 months and then routinely throughout their life.

According to the CDC, "Following the 5th dose – at least 9 out of 10 kids are fully protected" (CDC, 2019). I would like to point out that it already falls short of the 95% of the population needed to prevent the spread of the disease and it took 5 doses to get there. Then the CDC website goes on to say, "There is a modest decrease in effectiveness in each following year. About 7 out of 10 kids are fully protected 5 years after getting their last dose of DTaP."

Tdap, which is the adult version of the DTaP vaccine, will protect "7 out of 10 people who receive it. There is a decrease in effectiveness in each following year. About 3 or 4 out of 10 people are fully protected 4 years after getting Tdap" (CDC, 2019). The Tdap vaccine for adults is only recommended once every 10 years for the general public! With these rates, there is absolutely no way to ever achieve herd immunity, thus completely devaluing the idea of herd immunity for mandatory vaccination.

Third, herd immunity assumes vaccines prevent the transmission of the disease. A very common argument for mass vaccination against Pertussis is herd immunity. However, the FDA released a document stating: "This research suggests that although individuals immunized with an acellular pertussis vaccine may be protected from disease, they may still become infected with the bacteria without always getting sick and are able to spread infection to others, including young infants who are susceptible to pertussis disease" (Infection Control Today, 2013).

Studies show that even if a vaccine doesn't stop you from getting the disease (vaccine failure), the symptoms will be milder (Deiss et al., 2015). This is beneficial for the person who has milder chickenpox (Mayo Clinic, n.d.) or has less of a cough with pertussis (CDC, 2019), but does this actually protect the herd? A stronger argument might be that it would actually put the herd at greater risk by spreading diseases we don't actually know we have.

Lastly, it provokes the question, are we putting immunocompromised people at greater risk of disease if many individuals are actually infected with the disease but not showing symptoms? One of the first things people learn when immunocompromised is to stay away from anyone showing any sign of disease. However, if an infected person is not showing signs of disease, the immunocompromised individual will not know they need to avoid that person, thereby putting them at an increased risk of disease contraction.

Protecting the herd is always going to be the goal of the government and its regulating bodies. However, it must also be mentioned that we should never sacrifice an individual for the sake of the herd. No parent should be forced into a decision that could result in the death or injury of their child to protect the idea of the greater good. Every life matters. Every person should get to consider their personal history and perform their own risk assessment before consenting to a procedure. It is noble to "get the flu shot to protect others," but what does that mean to the parents that lost their children while trying to protect yours. Is your life more valuable?

Chapter 7
Informed Consent

In all aspects of medicine, informed consent is the pillar on which all medical interventions stand. Providers are legally obligated to inform patients of the risks and benefits of having or not having an intervention or treatment. Without informed consent, an intervention is essentially an assault.

It is tough to find individuals who are even willing to entertain a discussion about vaccinations. This is systematically problematic. Advances in medicine are made daily, information is more readily available now than ever before, and our approaches to medicine should be dynamic enough to reflect our knowledge base at that time. We do the best with the information we have at a given time. With that being considered, there is always room to learn more. Discussions are a great way to explore new ideas and learn about the research you may not have been exposed to before. One of two things happen with continued knowledge: 1) we solidify our current belief system or 2) we are enlightened to explore new information and ways of thinking. In either scenario, we are open and humble enough to continue to grow.

Ask yourself this, if you have been vaccinated, can you name three adverse reactions to any of the vaccinations you have received? Were you told what the risks were if you abstained from getting the vaccine? Were you told the efficacy rates of getting it? These are all important components that need to be understood in order to make an informed choice.

According to the Centers for Disease Control and Preventions Morbidity and Mortality Weekly Report (Flannery et al., 2018), "VE [Vaccine Efficacy] point estimates against medically attended influenza for all virus types varied by age group; statistically significant protection against medically attended influenza was found among children aged 6 months through 8 years (VE = 59%; CI = 44%–69%) and adults aged 18–49 years (VE = 33%; CI = 16%–47%), whereas no statistically significant protection was observed in other age groups."

Children age 9-17 and adults ages 50+ had no measurable benefit from getting the flu vaccine. That means anyone who received the vaccination in those age ranges would derive no benefit but still face the known risk. The risk factors, according to the Table of Injuries, are Guillain-Barré Syndrome, vasovagal syncope, anaphylaxis, and shoulder injury related to vaccine administration.

If you are over the age of 65 and received the flu vaccine in the 2017-2018 flu season, the following information would have been very helpful in deciding if the flu vaccine was appropriate for you. According to the package insert provided by the manufacturer: "In adults 65 years of age and older, the most common

(≥10%) injection site reaction was pain (33%); the most common solicited systemic adverse reactions were myalgia (18%), headache (13%), and malaise (11%)." Knowing this, do you think the recommendation is appropriate for everyone? Being informed is essential in making appropriate healthcare decisions and the responsibility should be in the hands of providers offering them. The last time I went to Target for a vaccine, I don't remember hearing about any side effects, but I do remember the coupon for 10% off my purchase.

Chapter 8
Compulsory Vaccination

The opposite end of the spectrum to informed consent is compulsory vaccination. In 2019, five states (California, Mississippi, Maine, New York, and West Virginia) implemented compulsory vaccination as a prerequisite for children if they want to attend public or private schools and child care centers. This means that the only way for parents to avoid vaccination is through a medical exemption. You may NOT choose a personal or religious belief exemption. This goes way beyond the argument between "pro-vax" and "anti-vax."

Regardless of where you fall on the spectrum of vaccinations, everyone should be concerned about compulsory vaccination. No medical interventions for an individual should be subject to a community vote or mandate from elected representatives. There is no medical intervention that is safe and effective for everyone and therefore every medical intervention should be the right of the individual. We know vaccines have risks, which is why there is a tax on them to pay for their injuries. That being said, the government does not and should not have control over your or your child's body.

Consider this, according to the CDC's recommended vaccine schedule, infants should receive the Hepatitis B vaccine on the first day of life, usually within a few hours of being born. On this schedule, a provider has no time to understand the complete health picture of a child and therefore it would be impossible to predict if that child is a good candidate for that vaccination. In addition to this, Hepatitis B is commonly a sexually transmitted disease (or spread through needle sharing). No infant should or would be engaging in these activities; therefore, making the vaccine useless at that point. The child is undergoing risks for no known benefit at that time.

Additionally, the Hepatitis B vaccine contains 250 mcg of aluminum, which has been shown to have significant health consequences with ingestion. The Food and Drug Administration (FDA) has created a "safe does of aluminum" based on weight at 5 mcg per kilogram of body weight (Poole et al., 2011). Let's say a baby weighs 5 kilos, which is an 11 lb. baby, the safe dose would be 25 mcg, making the vaccine dose 10x the FDA safe limit. According to the Material Safety Data Sheet (MSDS):

> Chronic ingestion of aluminum may cause Aluminum Related Bone Disease or aluminum-induced Osteomalacia with fracturing Osteodystrophy, microcytic anemia, weakness, fatigue, visual and auditory hallucinations, memory loss, speech and language impairment (dysarthria, stuttering, stammering, anomia, hypofluency, aphasia and eventually, mutism), epileptic seizures(focal or grand mal), motor disturbance(tremors, myoclonic jerks, ataxia, convulsions, asterixis, motor apraxia, muscle fa-

tigue), and dementia (personality changes, altered mood, depression, diminished alertness, lethargy, 'clouding of the sensorium', intellectual deterioration, obtundation, coma), and altered EEG. (The Human Metabolome Database, 2012)

One dose may not qualify as chronic exposure but the risk must be considered seeing that aluminum is in the following vaccines: DTaP, Tdap, Pneumococcal, human papillomavirus (HPV), hepatitis A, hepatitis B, haemophilus influenzae type b (Hib), inactivated polio vaccine (IPV), and Influenza. All of these vaccines make up a large portion of the AT LEAST 54 doses a child receives before the age of 18.

Furthermore, animal studies have shown that aluminum does cross the blood-brain barrier (Sharma, Hussain, Schlager, Ali, & Sharma, 2009) and human studies and autopsies are showing that aluminum can contribute to the development of Alzheimer's. The blood-brain barrier is a unique system designed to protect the central nervous system from toxins, pathogens, inflammation, injury, and disease. It is a safeguard the body has created to help keep us healthy when exposed to dangerous substances. Scientists are now recommending that "immediate steps should be taken to lessen human exposure to Al [aluminum], which may be the single most aggravating and avoidable factor related to AD [Alzheimer's disease]" (Tomljenovic, 2011).

Moreover, there are strong financial incentives for this particular medical intervention for both the patient and the provider. The individuals recommending and administering the vaccinations get a financial kickback from insurance companies if enough of their patient population is fully vaccinated. Individuals receive discounts on groceries or free giveaways for being vaccine compliant. To further simplify this, the government is mandating that infants get injected with a known toxic substance at 10x their own safe limit on the first day of life for a disease that the likelihood of getting is next to zero!

Lastly, in 1948 the United Nations wrote The Universal Declaration on Human Rights, which established access to education as a basic human right. Children who are not vaccinated in compliance with school immunization requirements are not permitted to enter school without a medical exemption.

Just go get a medical exemption would be the easy answer, right? Wrong! Physicians who are writing medical exemptions are being personally targeted and threatened by the medical board. After SB 276 passed in California in 2019, the criteria for obtaining a medical exemption were removed from the pediatrician and placed solely in the hands of the state. Every time a doctor decides a child needs a medical exemption, it must be in accordance with the reasons set forth by the state. All medical exemptions will be reviewed by a state official, not a medical doctor, and then it will be determined if it is valid. These officials will never meet the child, yet they hold the power of their medical freedom.

Chapter 9
SB276 Of California –
The Suspected Implications

SB276 is a law that passed in California in 2019. It is important to understand that California is typically a launching ground for laws like SB276 and that these laws typically tend to spread through other democratic states. Under the new guidelines, which are still open to interpretation as implementation has not yet occurred, family history has been removed as a reason to avoid a specific vaccination.

A child must receive all vaccinations unless one of the few excusable reactions occurs. For example, your firstborn child receives the Varicella (chickenpox) vaccine and has an anaphylactic reaction and requires intensive medical care to recover, if they are lucky enough to survive. This is a known possible side effect as it is listed on the Table of Injuries and is paid for by the National Vaccine Injury Compensation Program, so it also should have been discussed as part of the informed consent.

Now you have a second child, they were born a little premature, have chronic digestive issues, eczema, and multiple food allergies but are still considered healthy. It is their first birthday, and now they are expected to get their first dose of the varicella vaccine. Would you do it? If you want them to attend daycare, public, private or a charter school, you have to.

Chapter 10
When Vaccines Fail To Protect The Public

Vaccines are administered for the basic idea of protecting the population from communicable diseases. When they fail, and an outbreak occurs, the vaccine is never to blame, it is the percentage of the population that did not utilize the vaccination that gets blamed.

It's not failure to vaccinate, it's vaccine failure. The manufacturer of the mumps vaccine is currently under investigation for falsifying data claims of efficacy after two former Merck (a vaccine manufacturing company) employees filed a lawsuit against them (Chatom Primary Care, P.C. v. Merck & Co., Inc., 2012). There is a threshold of efficacy that must be met in clinical trials for the vaccine to be considered for the market. There is strong evidence that the data was manipulated to appear more efficacious. In fact, there have been quite a few mumps outbreaks over the past few years in populations with 100% vaccination rates.

There is the U.S. Navy ship that was stuck at sea for almost 4 months because it was being quarantined for a mumps outbreak on the ship. Our military is subject to compulsory vaccination, yet the outbreak still occurred. Second, in 2019, 67 cases of mumps were tied to the Temple University outbreak, yet Temple University requires 2 doses of the measles, mumps, and rubella (MMR) vaccine prior to attendance.

Lastly, the Disneyland measles outbreak in 2015 was the catalyst for SB277, which removed both religious and personal belief exemptions for individuals in California. However, according to the *Journal Clinical Microbiology*, "Of the 194 measles virus sequences obtained in the United States in 2015, 73 were identified as vaccine sequences" (Roy et al., 2017). This means that the vaccine caused almost 38% of the cases, presumably through viral shedding. Vaccines do have the ability to cause the disease they are trying to prevent so it is very important to distinguish between wild strains and vaccine strains when looking at suspected outbreaks.

Again, I am not saying that no one should have vaccinations if they choose, I am pointing out the fact that the benefits may be overstated while the risks are often understated. And above all else, that it should be up to the individual or guardian to make that decision.

Chapter 11
Food For Thought

The HPV vaccine is under consideration to be added to the required vaccination schedule in New York for entry to school. This is interesting as HPV is not spread through close contact and therefore is not a threat to the community or herd in the same way as pertussis or influenza. The vaccine was created to prevent certain cancers in the individual, not to protect the community. Additionally, there are some interesting facts about HPV and the vaccine. Again, the point is not to stop you from getting the shot if you choose, I am just opening up the field to reasonable doubt and giving power back to parents and children to select which interventions they choose to undergo.

According to the package insert, 2.3% of study participants in safety trials reported having a serious adverse event. According to the NIH National Cancer Institute, approximately 0.6 percent of women will be diagnosed with cervical cancer at some point during their lifetime, based on 2014-2016 data (National Cancer Institute, n.d.). The rate of serious adverse events is over 3.5x the likelihood of developing cervical cancer. This also doesn't take into account the percentage of people who fully recover after diagnosis. Additionally, the HPV vaccines are being linked to impaired fertility. Women who have received the vaccination are less likely to conceive than their unvaccinated counterparts (DeLong, 2018).

Is it ethical to mandate a vaccine to protect against a condition that does not pose a communicable risk to the general population through normal societal interactions? Why should it be compulsory, seeing that it impacts a very low percentage of the population and is not spread through casual contact?

Chapter 12
Abortion And Vaccines

I am not starting a conversation on abortion, but it does directly affect the vaccine debate. According to a statement from the Vatican and multiple other sources, aborted fetuses are being used in the production of vaccines.

According to a 2018 research article, three vaccines utilize cell lines that were derived from fetal tissue harvested from elective abortions in the 1960s (McKenna, 2018). These cell lines can be found on the immunizations for rubella, varicella, or hepatitis A.

Additionally, the Vatican has released a lengthy document surrounding the use of aborted fetal cells in vaccines. Many individuals are not Catholic, but the statement does provide good information. A portion of the Position Statement from the Vatican reads:

> "To date, there are two human diploid cell lines which were originally prepared from tissues of aborted foetuses (in 1964 and 1970) and are used for the preparation of vaccines based on

live attenuated virus: the first one is the WI-38 line (Winstar Institute 38), with human diploid lung fibroblasts, coming from a female foetus that was aborted because the family felt they had too many children (G. Sven et al., 1969). It was prepared and developed by Leonard Hayflick in 1964 (L. Hayflick, 1965; G. Sven et al., 1969)[3] and bears the ATCC number CCL-75. WI-38 has been used for the preparation of the historical vaccine RA 27/3 against rubella (S.A. Plotkin et al., 1965)[4]. The second human cell line is MRC-5 (Medical Research Council 5) (human, lung, embryonic) (ATCC number CCL-171), with human lung fibroblasts coming from a 14 week male foetus aborted for "psychiatric reasons" from a 27 year old woman in the UK. MRC-5 was prepared and developed by J.P. Jacobs in 1966 (J.P. Jacobs et al., 1970)[5]. Other human cell lines have been developed for pharmaceutical needs, but are not involved in the vaccines actually available[6]" (Pontifical Academy for Life, n.d.).

The statement also mentions that certain Hepatitis A, Chickenpox, Polio, Rabies, and Smallpox vaccines were all prepared using human cell lines from aborted fetuses. For some, regardless of their specific religion, this information may create an ethical debate and therefore they should be allowed time to explore their thoughts on the subject prior to making a decision.

Dr. Stanley Plotkin, the developer of the Rubella vaccine and vaccine advocate, was interviewed under oath on January 11th, 2018. He confirmed in one of his research articles that 76 fetuses were used as "preparatory" to see if fetuses could be used in the creation of vaccines. He continued to confirm that all fetuses were three months or older, were normally developed, and were aborted for social and psychiatric reasons. Harvested tissues included skin, lung, heart, tongue, kidney, and spleen. Lastly, Dr. Plotkin admitted he had used orphans to study an experimental vaccine and that he could not deny using the mentally handicapped to study a vaccine.

This information represents a philosophical or moral objection to an intervention. It plays to the side of religion and ethics. But what if these do not pertain to you? Then I ask you this, should one have the right to bodily autonomy? Can a mom choose abortion if she sees fit? For many, the answer is yes. Pro-Choice is a large social decision, so I ask you to ponder why that should end because it is a needle instead of a scalpel. If one should be able to choose to get an abortion, one should be able to choose to abstain from vaccination.

Chapter 13
Has Science Proven Vaccines To Be Safe And Effective?

Science changes daily. Yes, there is some science that says the risk of vaccination is less than the risk of acquiring that specific communicable disease. There are also substantial resources proving vaccines cause a lot of injury and harm.

We have proven that chemotherapy is effective at treating many types of cancer. Saying that it is safe is relative. Chemotherapy has a known risk profile, cancer being one of its side effects. Interesting that a drug designed to treat cancer is also known to cause cancer. However, at this time, it is often considered the best tool we have available. That is a decision the patient gets to make. Also, because we have chemotherapy as a treatment option, it doesn't mean that we stop looking for new solutions or stop looking at its safety profile. That is how medicine progresses. We continually have people research, study, and discuss medical interventions to see if they are still the best option we have or if the risk is still worth the benefit. There should never be a time when we stop looking at safety!

Too often, the argument to vaccinate comes from parents who have been vaccine compliant and state, "my child was vaccinated and they're fine." This does not negate the fact that there are adverse reactions to vaccinations. In fact, when a child suffers from a vaccine-induced injury, parents are forced to join the "ex-vax" group, which immediately leads to them losing their reliability to the general public altogether.

Too many times parents believe what they want to believe—that they aren't endangering their child by following the CDC guidelines. The thought that they might subject their child to lifelong injury is too much to bear, so they become closed off to the conversation completely and refuse to be open to the opposing side. Too many times I have heard other mothers say, "I've done the research and vaccines are safe." But have they really done "research"? Or are they simply choosing to read information only supporting one side of the argument?

Something else to consider is what is the definition of "fine"? Does the fact that a child is alive mean that the vaccination didn't have any negative associated side effects? It is impossible to know how a child would grow and develop if they did/did not have a vaccination.

Chapter 14
Pregnancy and Vaccines

Two vaccines are currently recommended during pregnancy. They are the flu vaccine and the Tdap vaccine. If a woman's pregnancy spans over two flu seasons, then it is recommended that she receive it twice. In regard to vaccination during pregnancy, there are two very important points to address.

First, no vaccine has ever been tested for safety in pregnant women. This means that safety is assumed, but it has never been scientifically proven. As I mentioned before, we often hear the science is settled and vaccines are safe. In our arguably most vulnerable population, pregnant women, the science has never been conducted. Yes, there is an ethical implication of studying drugs on pregnant women, but there should also be an ethical consideration for injecting untested drugs in pregnant women especially with a drug that has a very low and transient efficacy rating.

Additionally, researchers discovered getting the flu vaccine during pregnancy increases the risk of miscarriage (Donahue et al., 2017). This reveals there are adverse reactions, including fetal death, from the vaccination. This should be incredibly alarming to parents and doctors, yet the information is often breezed over by the media. Today, so many families suffer from pregnancy loss. Having the choice, and at least all of the information regarding the lack of safety should be a top priority for all providers caring for this population. Unfortunately, this information is rarely shared.

There is a vaccine package insert that comes with every dose of vaccine, including the package insert for the flu vaccine administered during pregnancy. As I mentioned previously, it clearly states that safety and effectiveness have not been established in pregnant women. It continues to say there is a pregnancy registry available and to call Sanofi Pasteur Inc. at 1-800-822-2463.

In terms of post-market surveillance and discovering adverse reactions, it is very challenging as most individuals never are made aware of the pregnancy registry nor VAERS. Additionally, getting a vaccine during pregnancy and waiting to see fetal and pediatric development with so many additional variables is almost impossible. The absence of harm (or reports of harm) does not equate to the proof of safety. Taking a gamble on a population as vulnerable as pregnant moms is not a philosophy we should stand behind.

Chapter 15

Vaccinated Kids Playing With Unvaccinated Kids... Who Is At Risk?

Many parents say, "I don't want my kid playing with unvaccinated kids." This implies the unvaccinated kids are posing a bigger threat to society than vaccinated kids. Let's explore the flaws in this.

First, if you trust that vaccines are effective, an unvaccinated kid will pose no threat to a vaccinated child based on the belief that vaccines are effective. Consider this: if a child had measles and somehow exposed a vaccinated kid, then the vaccinated kid would be "immune" and therefore not be at risk. However, there *is* a risk to an unvaccinated kid being around a child recently vaccinated with the measles vaccine (MMR). Measles is a live virus vaccine and therefore can be spread through viral shedding.

Viral shedding is when the virus from a live vaccine is able to cause illness in another individual through secretions from the recently vaccinated individual. The CDC reports that it is very common in individuals following the Live Attenuated Influenza Vaccine (LAIV) (CDC, 2019). Vaccines can cause the disease they are trying to stop, not only in the vaccinated individual but in the individuals around them as well.

Additionally, people say it is the role of the children eligible for the vaccine to get it to protect the individuals who are not vaccine eligible. This goes back to protecting the herd. However, as previously explained, even if you have been vaccinated, you are still able to transmit the disease. You will not show as many symptoms and therefore are more likely to be around an immunocompromised individual because you don't know you are sick.

An unvaccinated individual will display signs and symptoms of the disease and be more likely to avoid the susceptible. Furthermore, many vaccine proponents state that vaccinations decrease the severity and the length of time they will suffer from a disease. That is for the betterment of that child, not the herd. Decreasing the severity would give an individual a false sense of wellbeing, placing immunocompromised individuals at greater risk again.

Lastly, the fear surrounding vaccine-preventable diseases has made people almost hysterical. People fear unvaccinated kids as if they are germ carriers of all diseases and playing with them will cause everyone around them to be exposed to all diseases. This is simply not true. Most children are healthy most of the time. And when we are not, our body has a unique way of telling us. From a rash to a fever to a cough, our body is showing us we are sick. This happens to both vaccinated and unvaccinated kids. All kids can spread disease! All kids can safely play when healthy. You cannot give a disease you do not have to someone else.

Chapter 16

My Pediatrician Will Not Keep Me As A Patient If I Refuse to Vaccinate

Currently, many pediatricians are denying care to patients who are not vaccinated. They state for the safety of their other patients, who must be vaccinated mind you, they are not willing to see patients who do not comply with the CDC schedule. However, they will happily see a patient who has pertussis, chickenpox or hepatitis B in their office as long as they were vaccinated and the vaccine just failed. These patients are just as likely to spread disease.

What if this became true for other procedures or diseases? What if hospitals stopped caring for young boys who were not circumcised? As health care providers, it is not our job to determine if someone is worthy of care, we provide it regardless of personal, religious, financial or philosophical differences because that is what is best for humanity.

This same level of discrimination has extended to schools. You cannot attend school if you don't have the hepatitis B vaccine, yet you can attend school if you are hepatitis B positive. There is a fear of discrimination against individuals who have a disease yet there is no light on the discrimination against individuals who decline medical interventions.

The reason pediatricians use for denying care is that they are following the guidelines from the American Academy of Pediatrics (AAP), which recommends following the CDC vaccination schedule as this dictates the Standard of Care. However, the AAP also has a position statement indicating that vaccine refusal should not be the reason for discharging a patient from a practice. The statement reads: "Continued refusal after adequate discussion should be respected unless the child is put at significant risk of serious harm (as, for example, might be the case during an epidemic)...In general, pediatricians should avoid discharging patients from their practices solely because a parent refuses to immunize his or her child" (Diekema, 2005).

It should also be noted that pediatricians are paid out their rates by insurance companies based on the percentage of their patient population that is fully vaccinated (BCBSRI, n.d.). We are talking tens of thousands to hundreds of thousands of dollars annually as long as they meet the benchmark. This places a huge incentive on physicians to vaccinate or not to see patients who do not comply as this can significantly impact their annual earnings.

It is a slippery slope in primary care to deny services based on differing opinions regarding certain medical interventions. Dentists don't stop seeing kids because some parents do or do not use fluoride. They educate on their perspective, high-light their training but fundamentally respect the wishes of the parent and child. Ultimately, everyone may learn something new by having open, honest, and well-researched conversations. If everyone in the world had the same opinions and viewpoints, progress would be forever stunted.

Chapter 17
Dr. Andrew Wakefield

If you have looked into the vaccine debate, I am sure you came across the name, Dr. Andrew Wakefield. Dr. Wakefield was a licensed medical doctor and a lead researcher on a paper published in the medical journal *Lancet* that was later retracted. As he is far from the main reason for vaccine hesitancy, I do not want to spend too much time rehashing the misdirected slander. However, I mention him because he has been disgraced by the media for the anti-vaccine movement. Many news articles will say that Dr. Wakefield claimed vaccines cause autism in his 1998 study published in the Lancet.

Three noteworthy points:

1. Dr. Wakefield was one of **thirteen authors** on the paper, yet no one else had punitive actions against them.
2. Vaccine hesitancy is not solely based on the fear of autism. Autoimmune conditions and other neurodegenerative conditions are the greatest reasons.
3. This is the conclusion of the study: "We have identified a chronic enterocolitis in children that may be related to neuropsychiatric dysfunction. In most cases,

the onset of symptoms was after measles, mumps, and rubella immunization. Further investigations are needed to examine this syndrome and its possible relation to this vaccine."

Dr. Wakefield never claimed that vaccines caused autism. The media portrayal of what happened was a gross misinterpretation designed to belittle individuals who are vaccine-hesitant. Even without any consideration for Dr. Wakefield, vaccine hesitancy would still be as strong as it is today.

Chapter 18
Are We Healthier?

With the expansion of the vaccine schedule, you would assume that our children would be getting healthier and that our country would be a hallmark for all other countries to aspire to. However, the U.S. has one of the worst infant mortality rates of industrialized nations, with 54 nations doing better (Central Intelligence Agency, n.d.). Despite our militant approach to vaccination, we still have way too many babies dying in the first year of life. Additionally, 54% of children today have a chronic disease, which is up from 12.8% in 1988 (Bethell et al., 2011; Van Cleave, Gortmaker, & Perrin, 2010).

Children in the U.S. are recommended to get at least 54 doses of vaccination by the age of 18 (CDC, 2019). In 1989, a child was recommended to have 12 doses to be considered up to date (Vaxopedia, 2019). There are 8-13 compulsory vaccines in the U.S. depending on which state you reside in (ProCon. org, 2018). Japan, by contrast, has no compulsory vaccines (Kuwabara & Ching, 2014). Japan also has the second-lowest infant mortality rate and the highest healthy life expectancy (EurekAlert, 2015). Monaco, the country with the lowest infant mortality rate, only requires three immunizations. Maybe we are missing the mark on our approach to keeping our children alive (Gouvernement Princier de Monaco, n.d.).

Chapter 19
Moving Forward

This information shared is not to start an argument, but rather to lay out some of the reasons for an educated decision. Take time to reflect on what you read and who, if someone other than yourself, wanted you to read it. Come to a discussion with an open mind, free of judgment, and with the intention of getting a better understanding of someone else's viewpoint. Discussions are not always meant to change somebody else's mind, but to hear somebody else's perspective. This is important to learn and grow both as individuals and as a society.

My hope is that one day vaccination discussions will be just that, a discussion. That individuals can be accepting of another approach to life and health. My hope is for a future full of health and freedom for all. My hope is that every parent has the right, power and knowledge to make the best decisions for their children and families. I see a future free of judgment, full of acceptance, and with the composure to handle challenging conversations with respect and tact.

I hope we can relinquish our views as the only truths and respect that life offers many paths.

"But just because I don't agree with someone on every-thing doesn't mean that I'm not going to be friends with them… When I say be kind to one another I don't mean only the people that think the same way that you do." ~ Ellen DeGeneres

References

BCBSRI. (n.d.). 2018 PCP Quality Incentive Program. Retrieved from https://www.bcbsri.com/sites/default/files/providers/pdf/BCBSRI-2018-PCP-Quality-Incentive-Program-Booklet_FINAL.pdf

Bethell, C. D., Kogan, M. D., Strickland, B. B., Schor, E. L., Robertson, J., & Newacheck, P. W. (2011). A National and State Profile of Leading Health Problems and Health Care Quality for US Children: Key Insurance Disparities and Across-State Variations. *Academic Pediatrics*, *11*(3), S22-S33. doi:10.1016/j.acap.2010.08.011

CDC. (2019). How the Flu Virus Can Change: "Drift" and "Shift". Retrieved from https://www.cdc.gov/flu/about/viruses/change.htm#targetText=One%20way%20influenza%20viruses%20change,)%20and%20NA%20(neuraminidase)

CDC. (2019). Pertussis Frequently Asked Questions. Retrieved from https://www.cdc.gov/pertussis/about/faqs.html

CDC. (2019). Safety of Influenza Vaccines. Retrieved from https://www.cdc.gov/flu/professionals/acip/safety-vaccines.htm

CDC. (2019). Birth-18 Years Immunization Schedule. Retrieved from https://www.cdc.gov/vaccines/schedules/hcp/imz/child-adolescent.html

Central Intelligence Agency. (n.d.). The World Factbook. Retrieved from https://www.cia.gov/library/publications/the-world-factbook/rankorder/2091rank.html

References

Chatom Primary Care, P.C. v. Merck & Co., Inc., 2:12-cv-03555 (2012).

Congress. (1986, October 14). H.R.5546 - National Childhood Vaccine Injury Act of 1986. Retrieved from https://www.congress.gov/bill/99th-congress/house-bill/5546

Deiss, R. G., Arnold, J. C., Chen, W., Echols, S., Fairchok, M. P., Schofield, C., ... Millar, E. V. (2015). Vaccine-associated reduction in symptom severity among patients with influenza A/H3N2 disease. *Vaccine, 33*(51), 7160-7167. doi:10.1016/j.vaccine.2015.11.004

DeLong, G. (2018). A lowered probability of pregnancy in females in the USA aged 25–29 who received a human papillomavirus vaccine injection. *Journal of Toxicology and Environmental Health, Part A, 81*(14), 661-674. doi:10.1080/15287394.2018.1477640

Diekema, D. S. (2005). Responding to Parental Refusals of Immunization of Children. *Pediatrics, 115*(5), 1428-1431. doi:10.1542/peds.2005-0316

Donahue, J. G., Kieke, B. A., King, J. P., DeStefano, F., Mascola, M. A., Irving, S. A., ... Belongia, E. A. (2017). Association of spontaneous abortion with receipt of inactivated influenza vaccine containing H1N1pdm09 in 2010-11 and 2011-12. *Vaccine, 35*(40), 5314-5322. doi:10.1016/j.vaccine.2017.06.069

EurekAlert. (2015). Life expectancy climbs worldwide but people spend more years living with illness and disability. Retrieved from https://www.eurekalert.org/pub_releases/2015-08/tl-lec082615.php

References

Flannery, B., Chung, J. R., Belongia, E. A., McLean, H. Q., Gaglani, M., Murthy, K., … Fry, A. M. (2018). Interim Estimates of 2017–18 Seasonal Influenza Vaccine Effectiveness — United States, February 2018. *MMWR Morb Mortal Wkly Rep 2018*, 67(6), 180–185.

Gouvernement Princier de Monaco. (n.d.). Vaccination schedule for children and teenagers. Retrieved from https://en.service-public-particuliers.gouv.mc/Social-health-and-families/Public-health/Prevention-and-screening/Vaccination-schedule-for-children-and-teenagers

Harris, G. (2009). Advisers on vaccines often have conflicts, report says. Retrieved from https://www.nytimes.com/2009/12/18/health/policy/18cdc.html

Health Resources & Services Administration. (2019). About the National Vaccine Injury Compensation Program. Retrieved from https://www.hrsa.gov/vaccine-compensation/about/index.html

Infection Control Today. (2013). FDA Study Helps Provide an Understanding of Rising Rates of Pertussis, Response to Vaccination. Retrieved from https://www.infectioncontroltoday.com/infectious-diseases-conditions/fda-study-helps-provide-understanding-rising-rates-pertussis-response

Kuwabara, N., & Ching, M. S. (2014). A Review of Factors Affecting Vaccine Preventable Disease in Japan. *Hawaii J Med Public Health*, 73(12), 376–381.

Mayo Clinic. (n.d.). Chickenpox. Retrieved from https://www.mayoclinic.org/diseases-conditions/chickenpox/symptoms-causes/syc-20351282

McKenna, K. C. (2018). Use of Aborted Fetal Tissue in Vaccines and Medical Research Obscures the Value of All Human Life. *The Linacre Quarterly, 85*(1), 13-17. doi:10.1177/0024363918761715

Mikulic, M. (2019). Total vaccine market revenues worldwide. Retrieved from https://www.statista.com/statistics/265102/revenues-in-the-global-vaccine-market/

National Cancer Institute. (n.d.). Cancer Stat Facts: Cervical Cancer. Retrieved from https://seer.cancer.gov/statfacts/html/cervix.html

Offit, P. A. (2019, December 18). *Vaccine History: Developments by Year*. Retrieved from https://www.chop.edu/centers-programs/vaccine-education-center/vaccine-history/developments-by-year

Pontifical Academy for Life. (n.d.). Moral reflections on vaccines prepared from cells derived from aborted human foetuses. Retrieved from https://www.immunize.org/talking-about-vaccines/vaticandocument.htm

Poole, R. L., Pieroni, K. P., Gaskari, S., Dixon, T. K., Park, K. T., & Kerner, J. A. (2011). Aluminum in Pediatric Parenteral Nutrition Products: Measured Versus Labeled Content. *J Pediatr Pharmacol Ther, 16*(2), 92–97. doi:10.5863/1551-6776-16.2.92

ProCon.org. (2018). State-by-State: Vaccinations Required for Public School Kindergarten. Retrieved from https://vaccines.procon.org/state-by-state-vaccinations-required-for-public-school-kindergarten/

Ross, L., & Klompas, M. (2011). *Electronic Support for Public Health–Vaccine Adverse Event Reporting System (ESP:VAERS)* (R18 HS 017045). U.S. Department of Health and Human Services.

References

Roy, F., Mendoza, L., Hiebert, J., McNall, R. J., Bankamp, B.,
Connolly, S., … Severini, A. (2017). Rapid Identification
of Measles Virus Vaccine Genotype by Real-Time
PCR. *Journal of Clinical Microbiology, 55*(3), 735-743.
doi:10.1128/jcm.01879-16

Sharma, H. S., Hussain, S., Schlager, J., Ali, S. F., &
Sharma, A. (2009). Influence of nanoparticles on
blood-brain barrier permeability and brain edema
formation in rats. *Acta Neurochir Suppl, 106*, 359-364.
doi:10.1007/978-3-211-98811-4_65

The Human Metabolome Database. (2012). Aluminum
MSDS. Retrieved from http://www.hmdb.ca/system/
metabolites/msds/000/001/116/original/HMDB01247.
pdf?1358893348

Tomljenovic, L. (2011). Aluminum and Alzheimer's Disease:
After a Century of Controversy, Is there a Plausible
Link? *Journal of Alzheimer's Disease, 23*(4), 567-598.
doi:10.3233/jad-2010-101494

Van Cleave, J., Gortmaker, S. L., & Perrin, J. M. (2010).
Dynamics of obesity and chronic health conditions
among children and youth. *JAMA, 303*(7), 623-630.
doi:10.1001/jama.2010.104

Vaxopedia. (2019). Historical Immunization Schedules.
Retrieved from https://vaxopedia.org/2016/10/26/
historical-immunization-schedules/